MY MS

AND ME

by Kevin Byrne

Illustrated by Nate Jensen

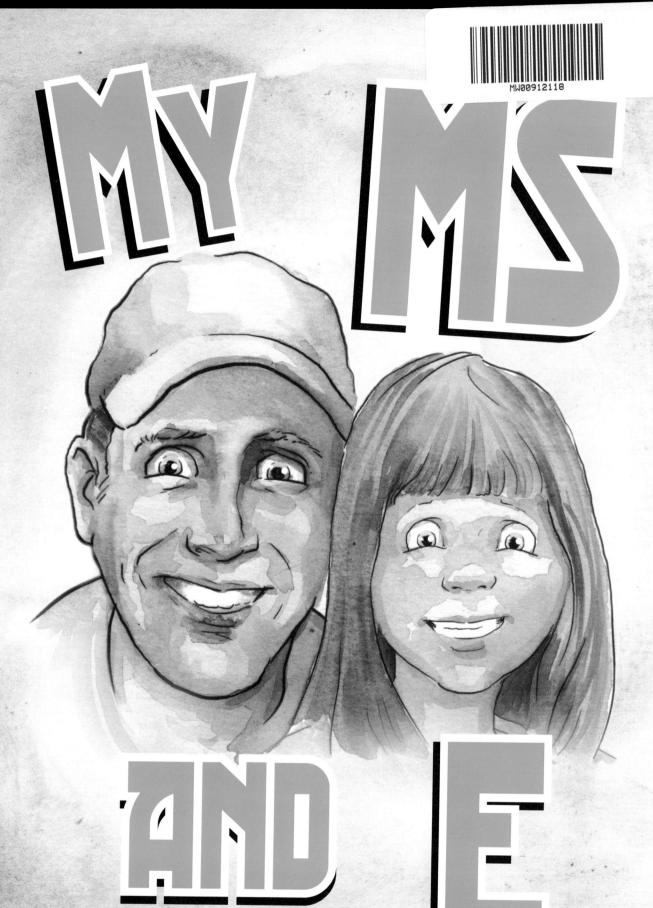

It is a fight.

For approximately 2.3 million people
with MS worldwide, the fight is not over
and it won't be over until the cure is found.

This book is dedicated to us,
our loved ones, and our supporters.
Thank you for the motivation every day.

It will never stop....nor will we
It will never quit....nor will we
This is why we ride.

Never Stop... Never Quit...®

Text © 2016 Kevin Byrne

Illustrations © 2016 Nathaniel P Jensen

Never Stop... Never Quit... Registered, U.S. Patent and Trademark Office

ISBN: 978-1-63491-592-2

Printed on acid-free paper.

The smile on the face
of our dear Eleanor
was a sight quite unlike
any seen there before!

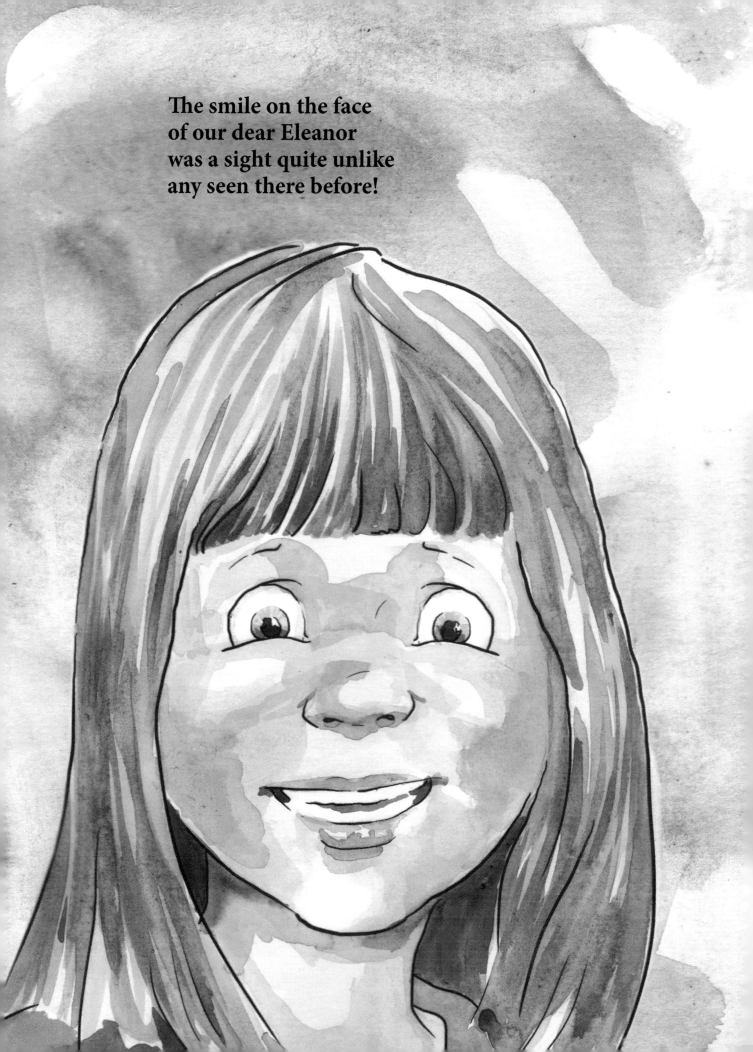

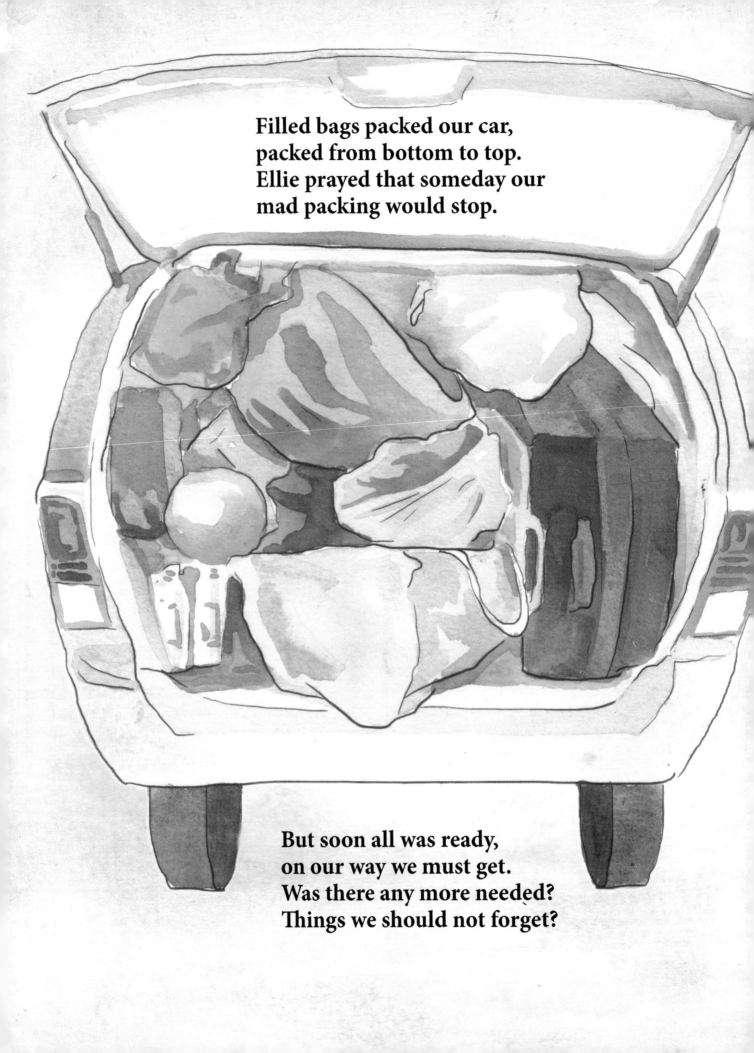

Filled bags packed our car,
packed from bottom to top.
Ellie prayed that someday our
mad packing would stop.

But soon all was ready,
on our way we must get.
Was there any more needed?
Things we should not forget?

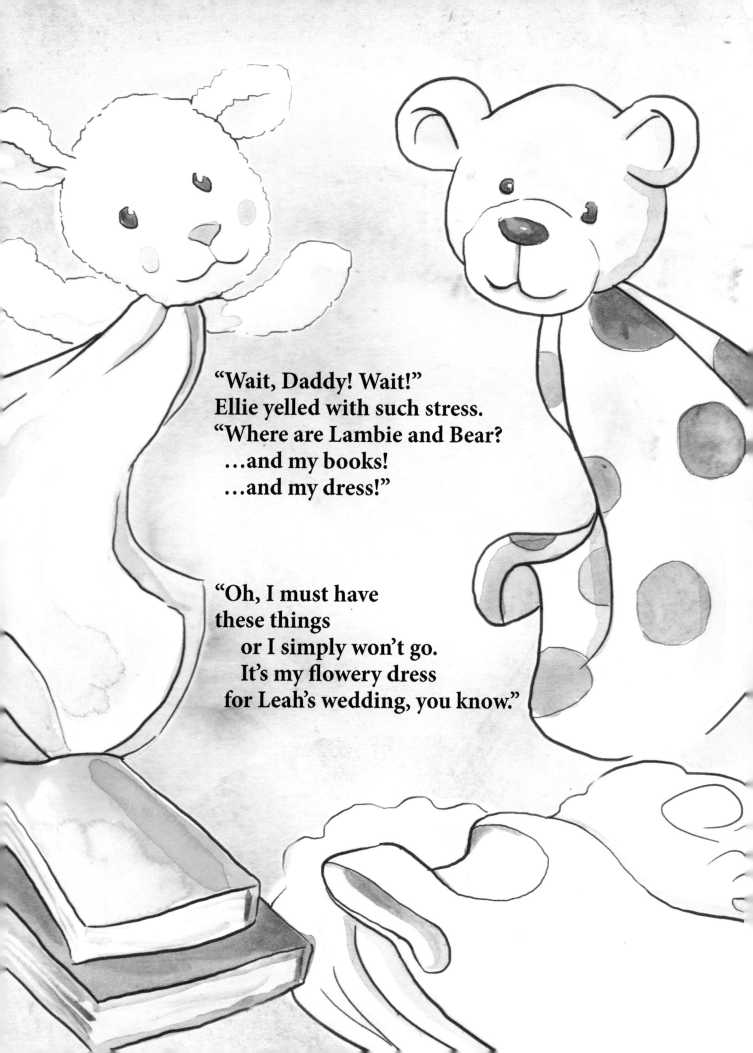

"Wait, Daddy! Wait!"
Ellie yelled with such stress.
"Where are Lambie and Bear?
 …and my books!
 …and my dress!"

"Oh, I must have
these things
   or I simply won't go.
   It's my flowery dress
 for Leah's wedding, you know."

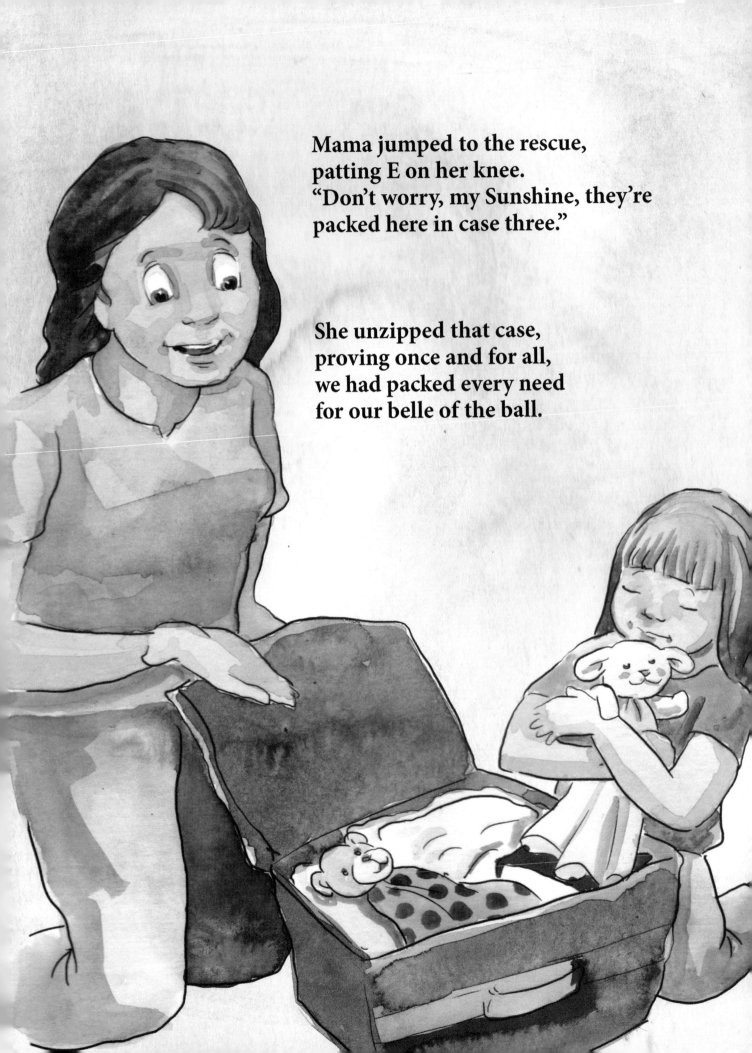

Mama jumped to the rescue,
patting E on her knee.
"Don't worry, my Sunshine, they're
packed here in case three."

She unzipped that case,
proving once and for all,
we had packed every need
for our belle of the ball.

So I climbed in my seat, with Brie close by my side.
We both turned to ensure E was ready to ride.

With that one final check, there was no more to do
except drive to Roche Harbor in a day, maybe two.

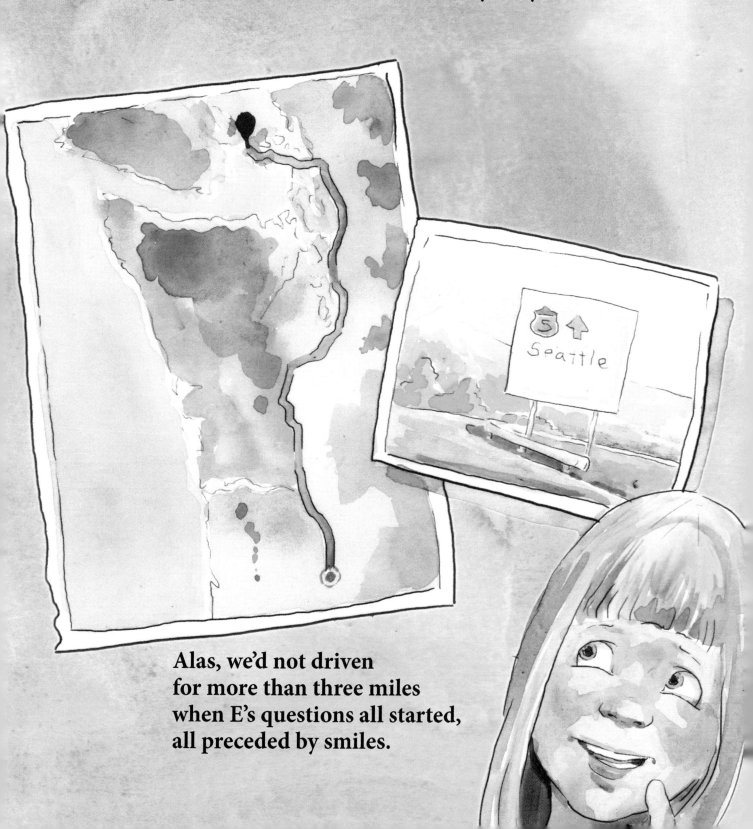

Alas, we'd not driven
for more than three miles
when E's questions all started,
all preceded by smiles.

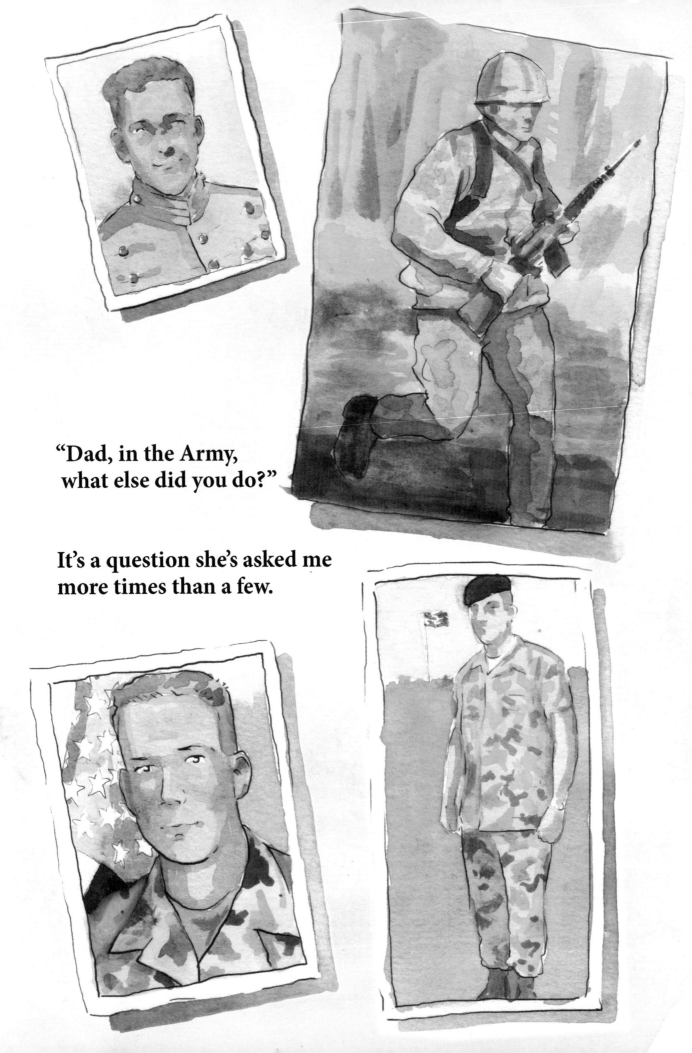

"Dad, in the Army,
what else did you do?"

It's a question she's asked me
more times than a few.

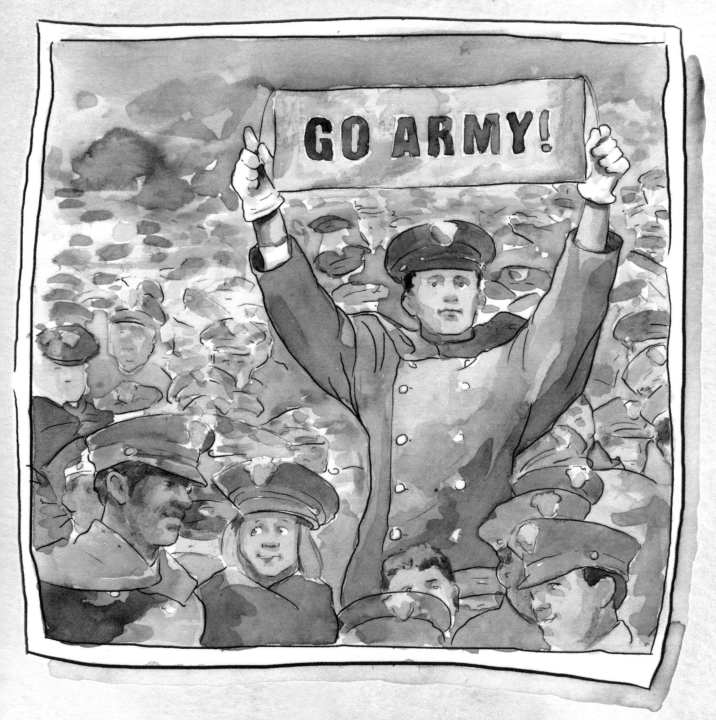

When E hears West Point cheers of
"Go Army! Beat Navy!"

She slyly replies,
"Yeah, Beat 'em. Beef Gravy!"

She knows "Ten minutes!
One minute! Stand in the door!"
Airborne School is a school E
would surely adore!

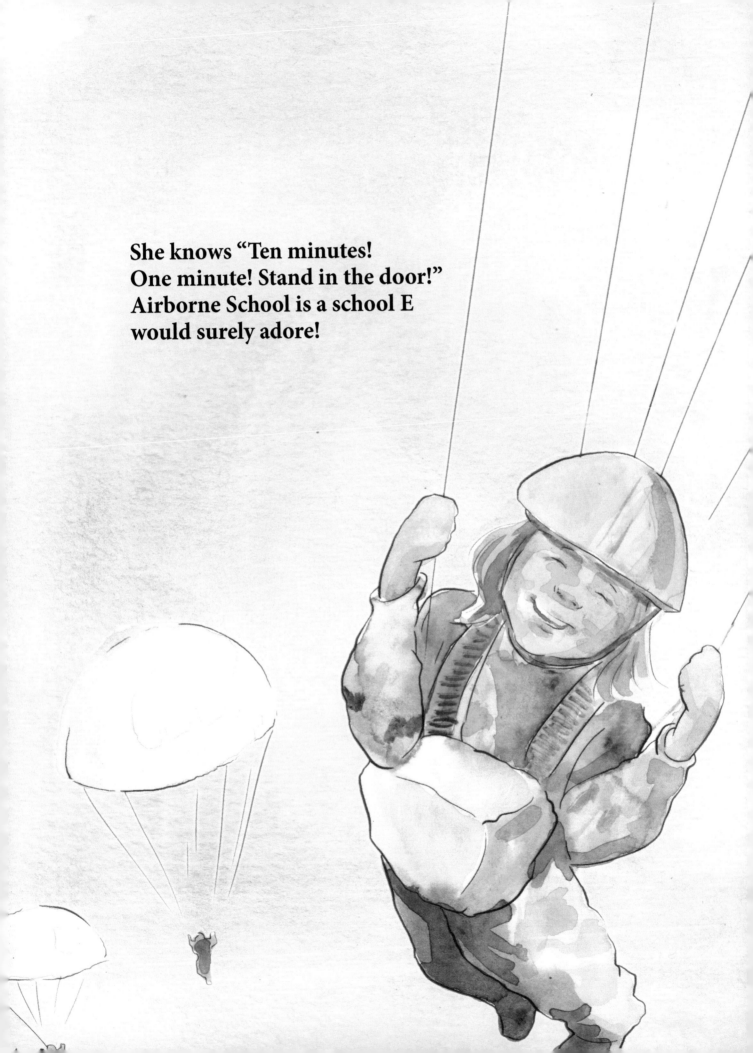

But I've started to run out of stories to use.
If I tell one I've told, E will simply refuse.

"Daddy, I know that. What else did you do?"
So I spin brand new tales,
    all exciting,
    all true.

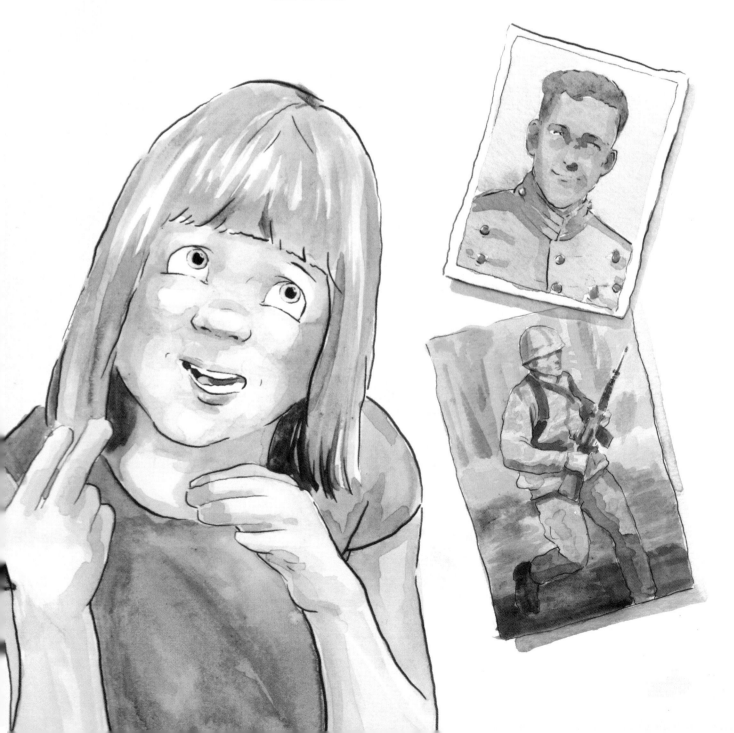

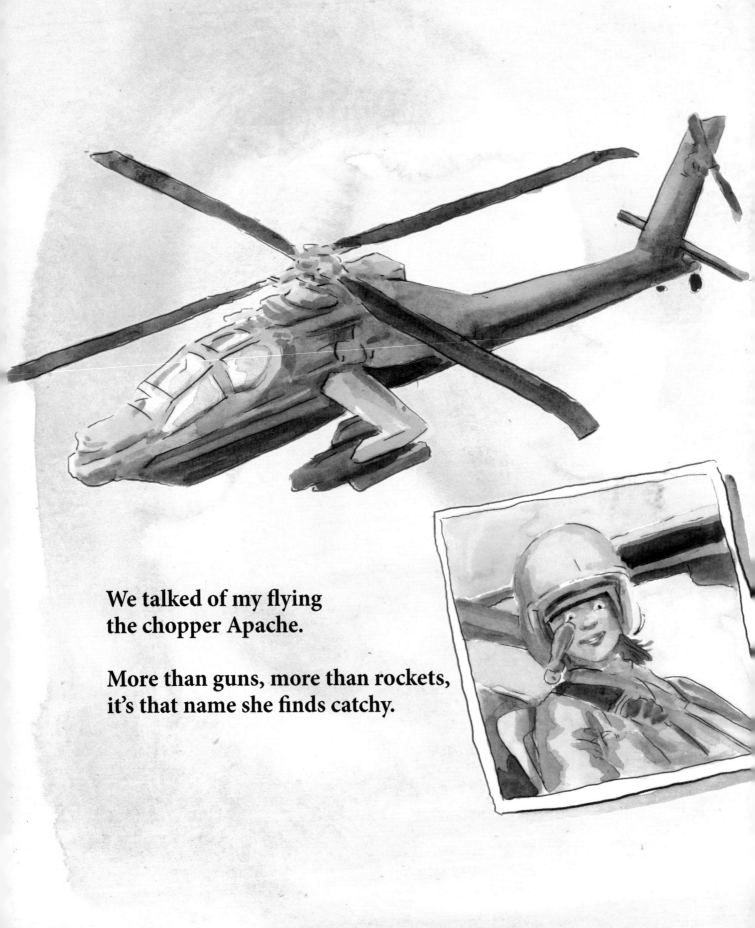

We talked of my flying
the chopper Apache.

More than guns, more than rockets,
it's that name she finds catchy.

"Why did you go Army? Will you ever go back?"
So I told E the tale of my MS attack.

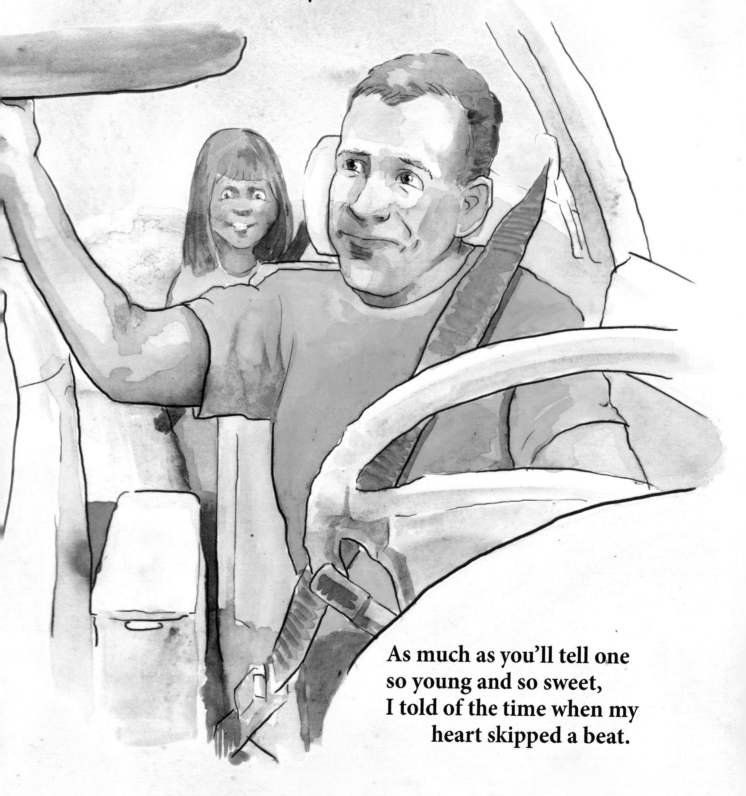

As much as you'll tell one
so young and so sweet,
I told of the time when my
heart skipped a beat.

With a tear in my eye I talked of those days
in a faraway land when I first heard that phrase.

I talked of those tests,
that start of my stress,
when a colonel declared simply,
"You have MS."

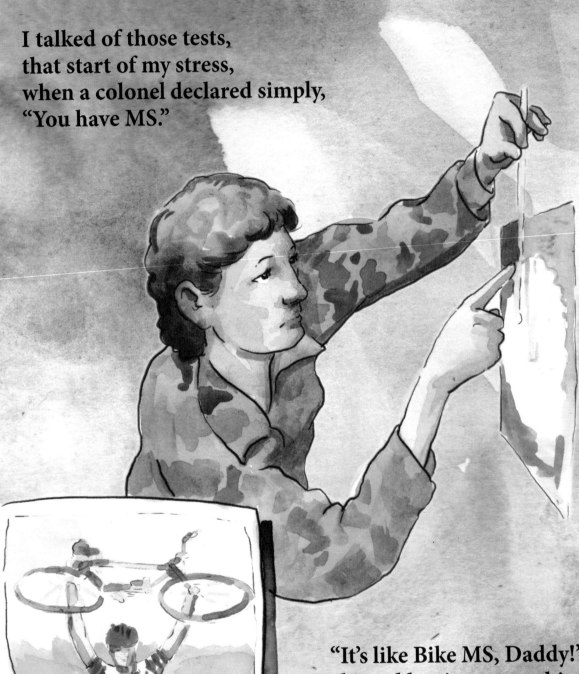

"It's like Bike MS, Daddy!"
chimed her innocent chimes.
For a part of E knows these
words only as rhymes.

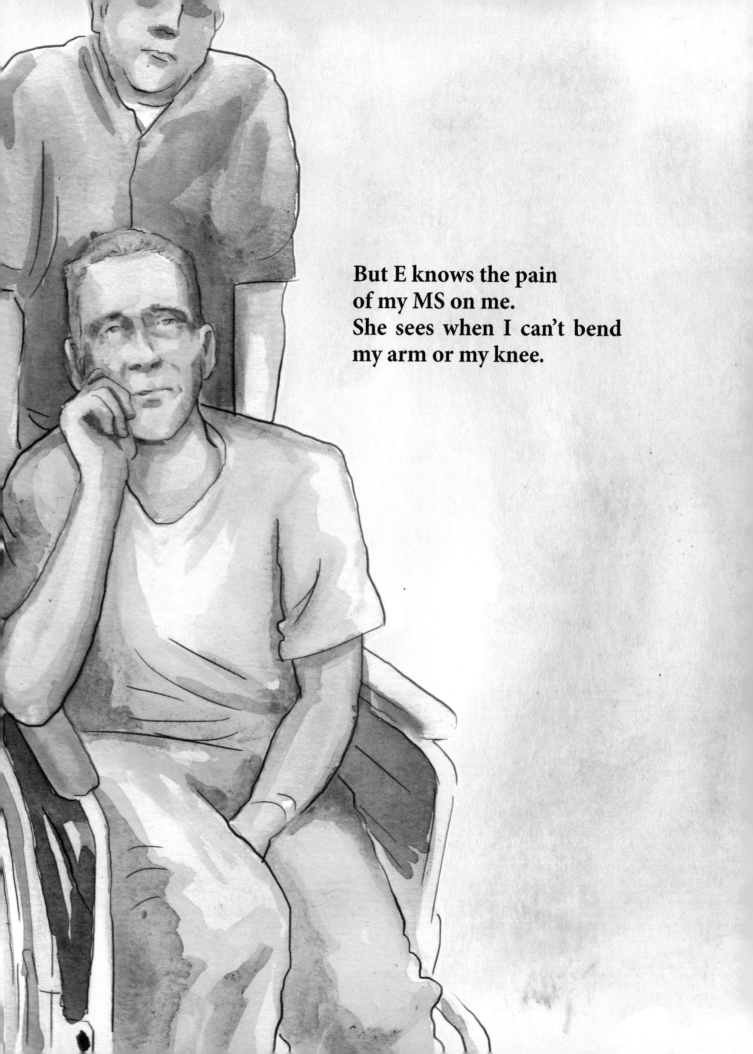

But E knows the pain
of my MS on me.
She sees when I can't bend
my arm or my knee.

My Eleanor knows there are
times I can't walk.
So we'll sit, just us two,
just to cuddle and talk.

And then, there are times
when my voice is so weak
no others will hear all the
words when I speak.

But E hears my words,
she hears what I say.
Yes, E understands,
even on my worst day.

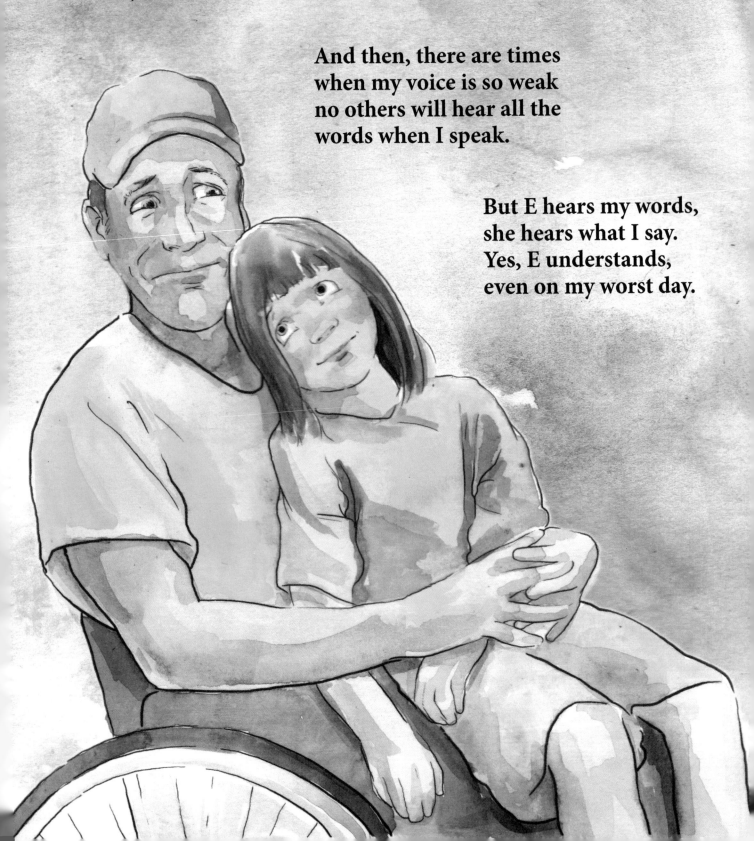

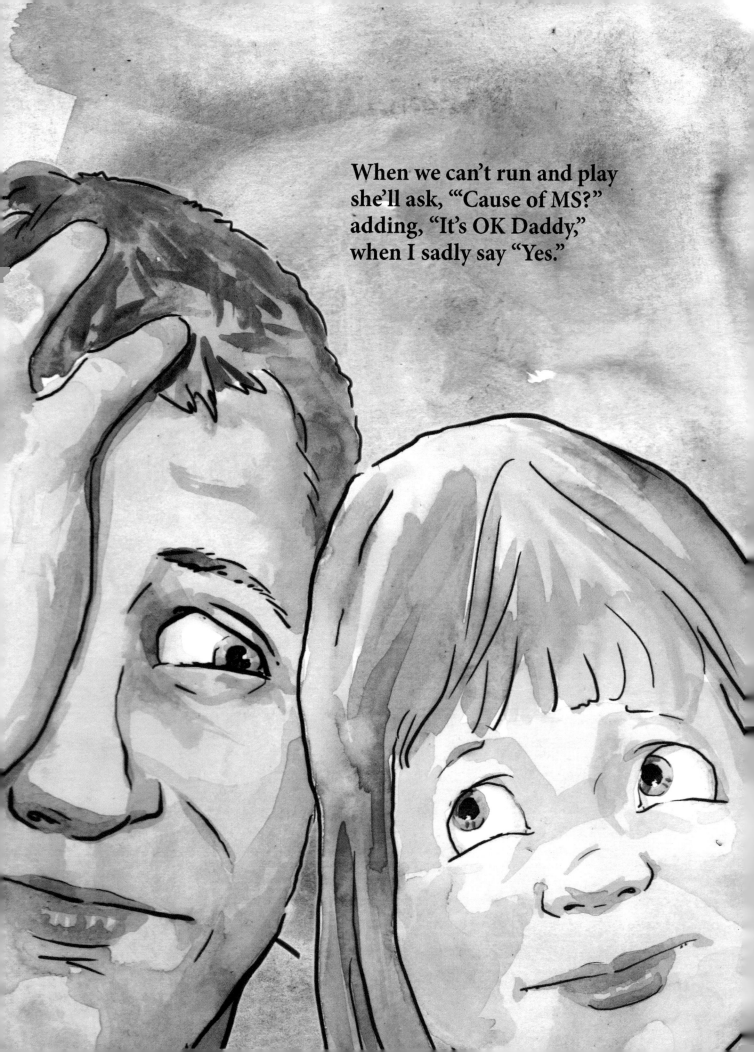

When we can't run and play
she'll ask, "'Cause of MS?"
adding, "It's OK Daddy,"
when I sadly say "Yes."

We talked of those days
before I was me.
But soon there were
sights more important
to see!

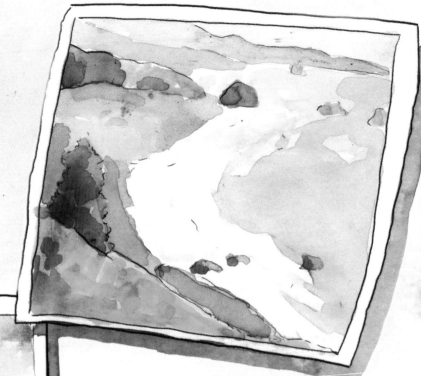

We drove down a highway.
We stopped for a night.
We rode on a ferry.
That was quite a delight!

We finally arrived
at the island resort.
For that drive,
when just five,
E was quite a good sport!

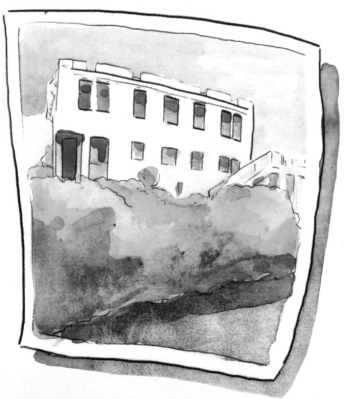

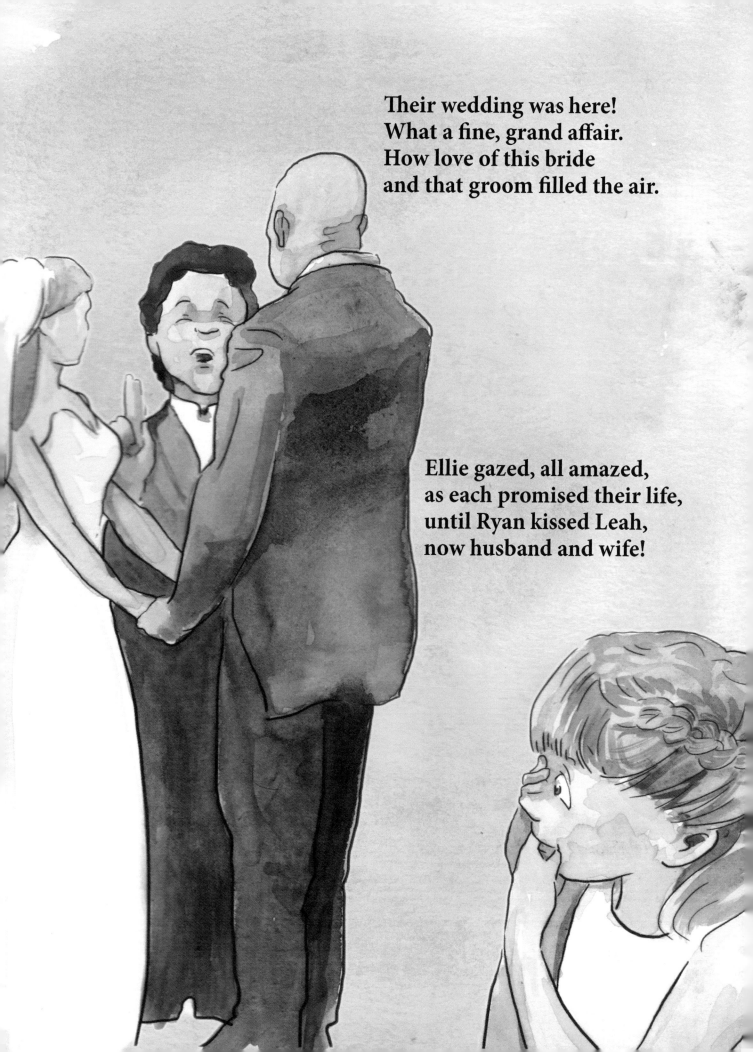

Their wedding was here!
What a fine, grand affair.
How love of this bride
and that groom filled the air.

Ellie gazed, all amazed,
as each promised their life,
until Ryan kissed Leah,
now husband and wife!

Then, after their vows,
came the party that night.
All the suits! All the dresses!
Every light shining bright.

All at once, Eleanor
saw she now had her chance.
When the Irish band played,
she exclaimed,
"Now, let's dance!"

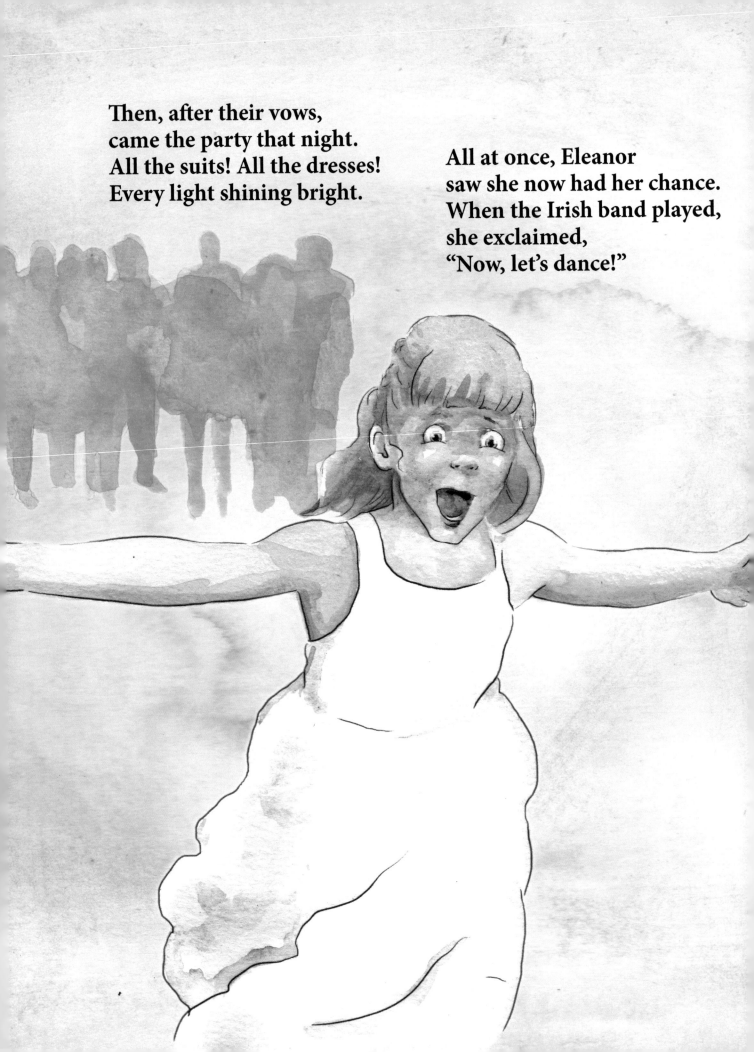

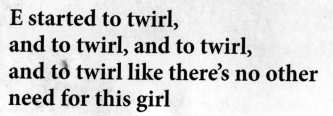

E started to twirl,
and to twirl, and to twirl,
and to twirl like there's no other
need for this girl

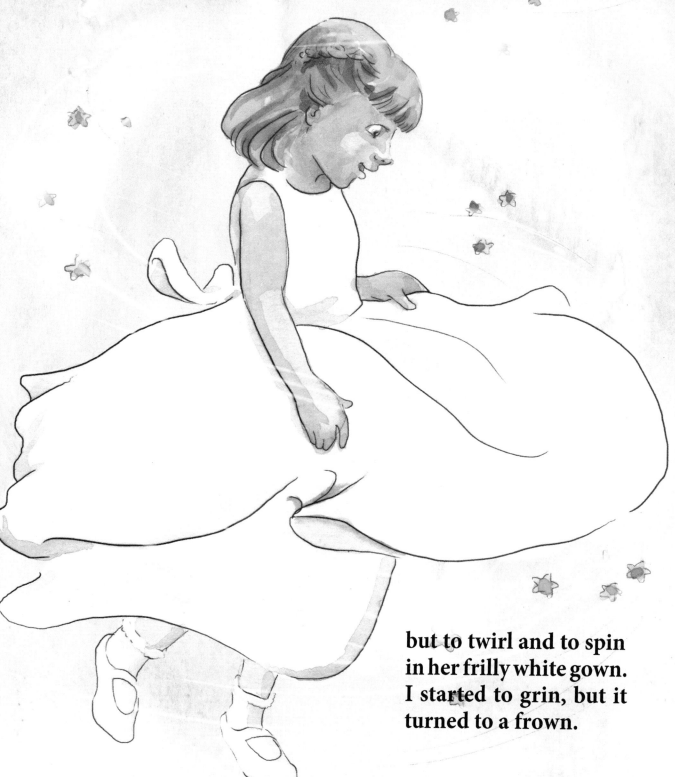

but to twirl and to spin
in her frilly white gown.
I started to grin, but it
turned to a frown.

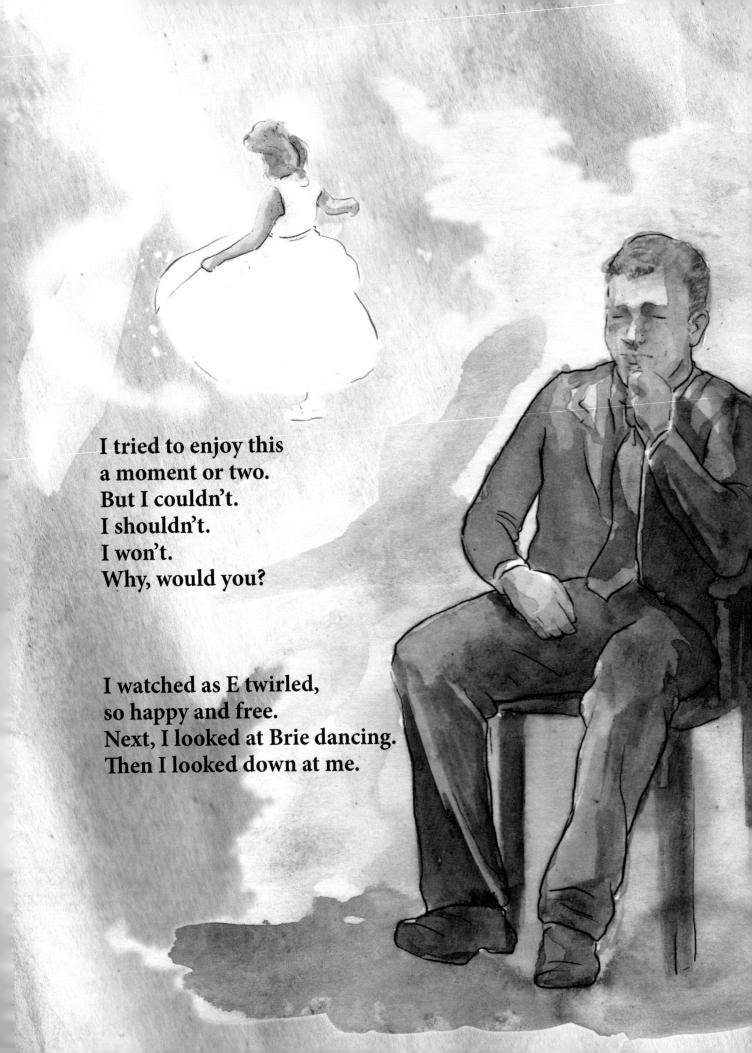

I tried to enjoy this
a moment or two.
But I couldn't.
I shouldn't.
I won't.
Why, would you?

I watched as E twirled,
so happy and free.
Next, I looked at Brie dancing.
Then I looked down at me.

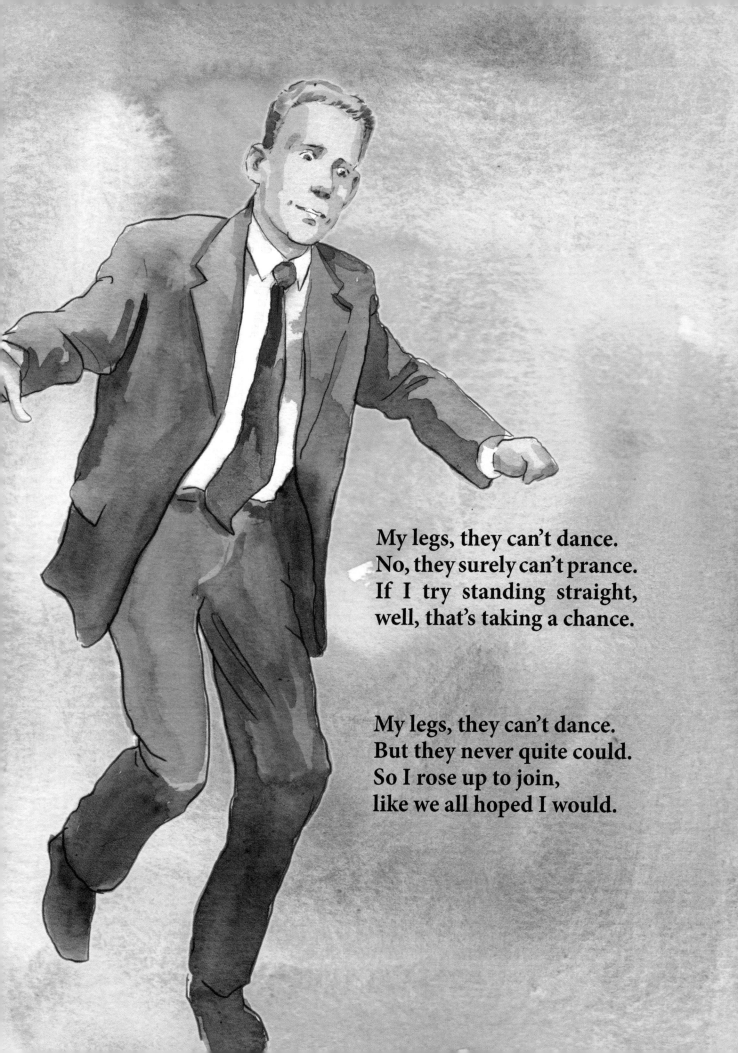

My legs, they can't dance.
No, they surely can't prance.
If I try standing straight,
well, that's taking a chance.

My legs, they can't dance.
But they never quite could.
So I rose up to join,
like we all hoped I would.

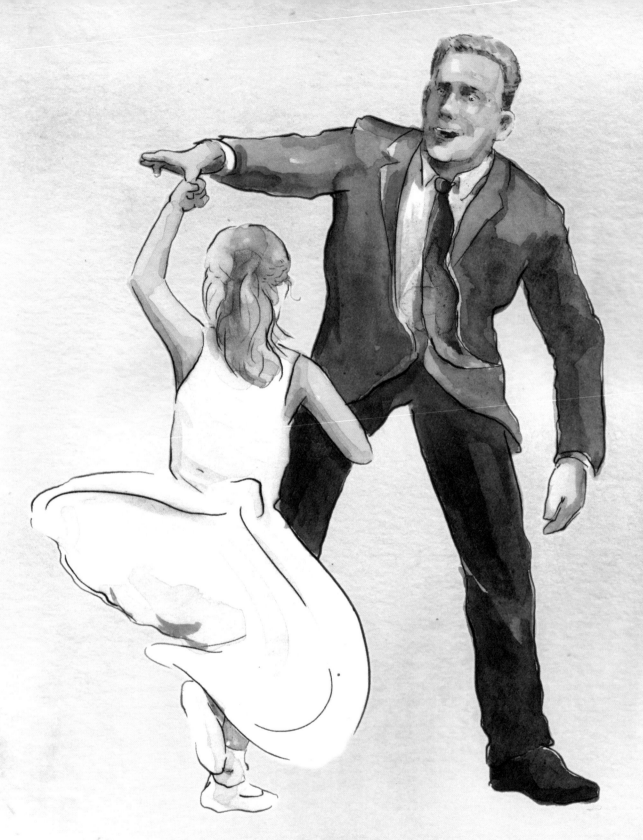

Well, I stumbled and bumbled
and limped 'cross the floor.
We all laughed as we danced
like we've never before.

First, "Daddy, be careful,"
warned worrisome E.
Soon, "Dance now with Mama!"
Then, "Now twirl with me!"

Ellie showed grave concern
when I spun my first spin.

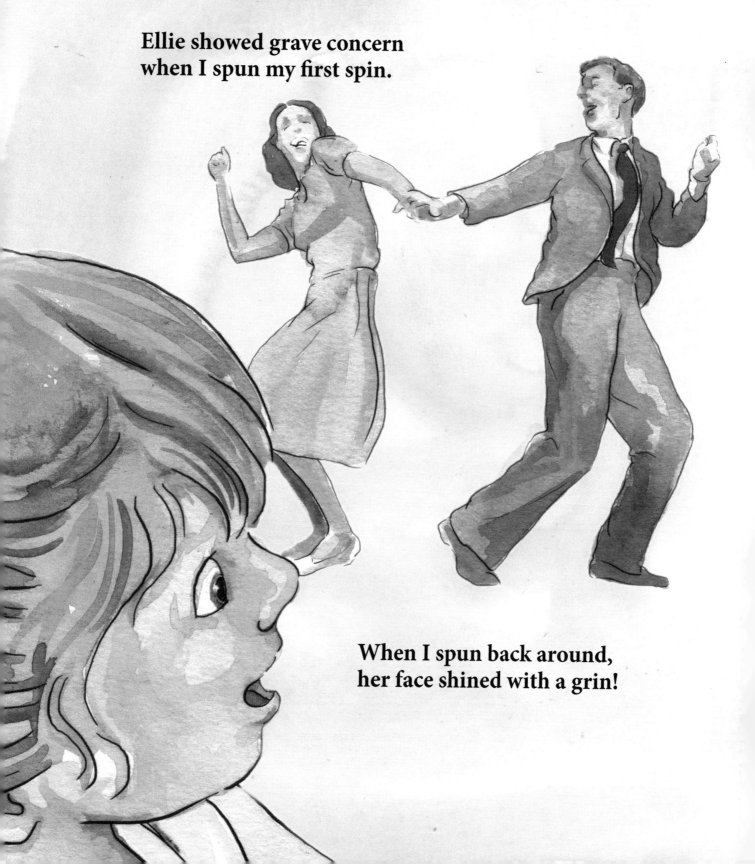

When I spun back around,
her face shined with a grin!

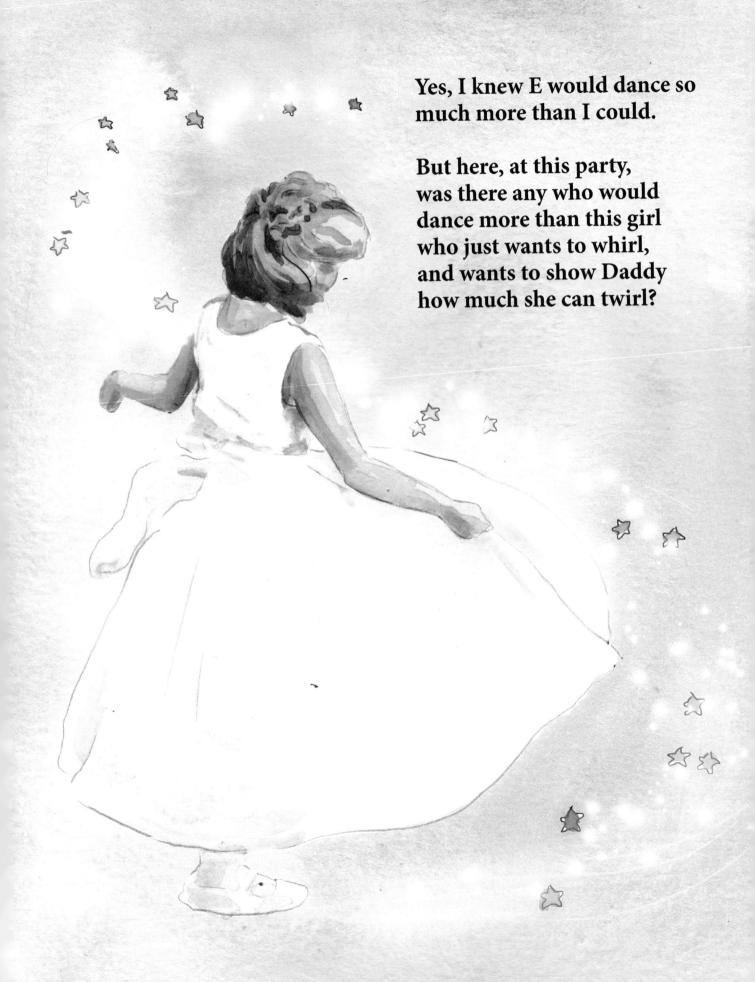

Yes, I knew E would dance so much more than I could.

But here, at this party, was there any who would dance more than this girl who just wants to whirl, and wants to show Daddy how much she can twirl?

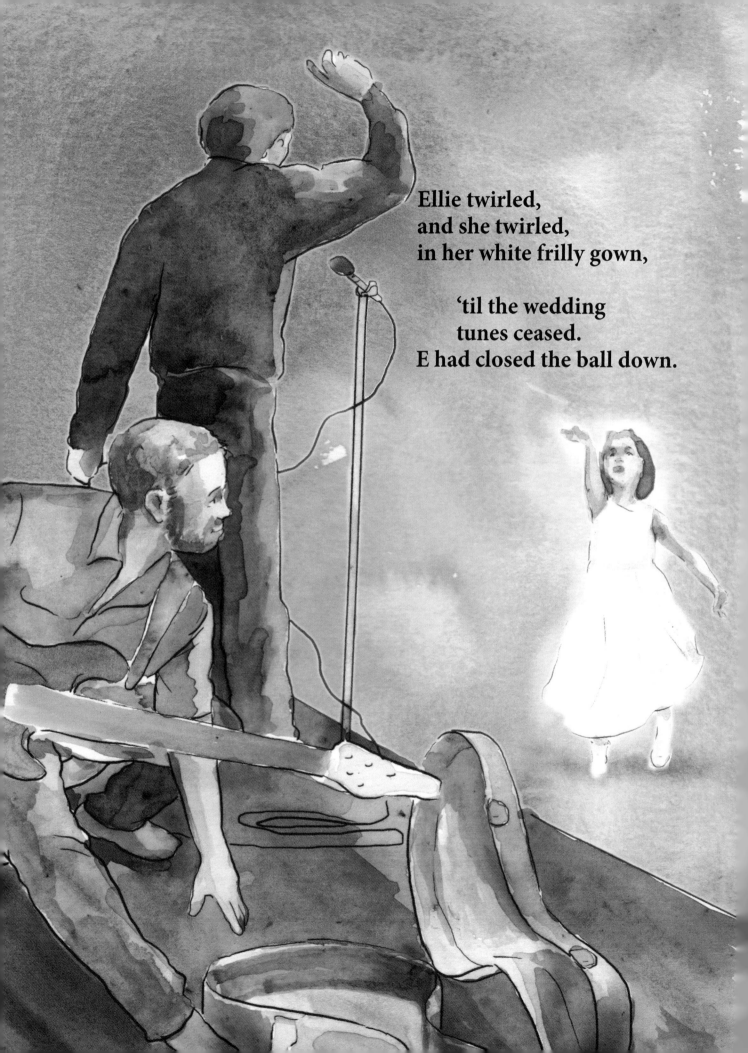

Ellie twirled,
and she twirled,
in her white frilly gown,

'til the wedding
tunes ceased.
E had closed the ball down.

After five fun-filled days
with fond memories to keep,
we drove back to Portland
for a night of good sleep.

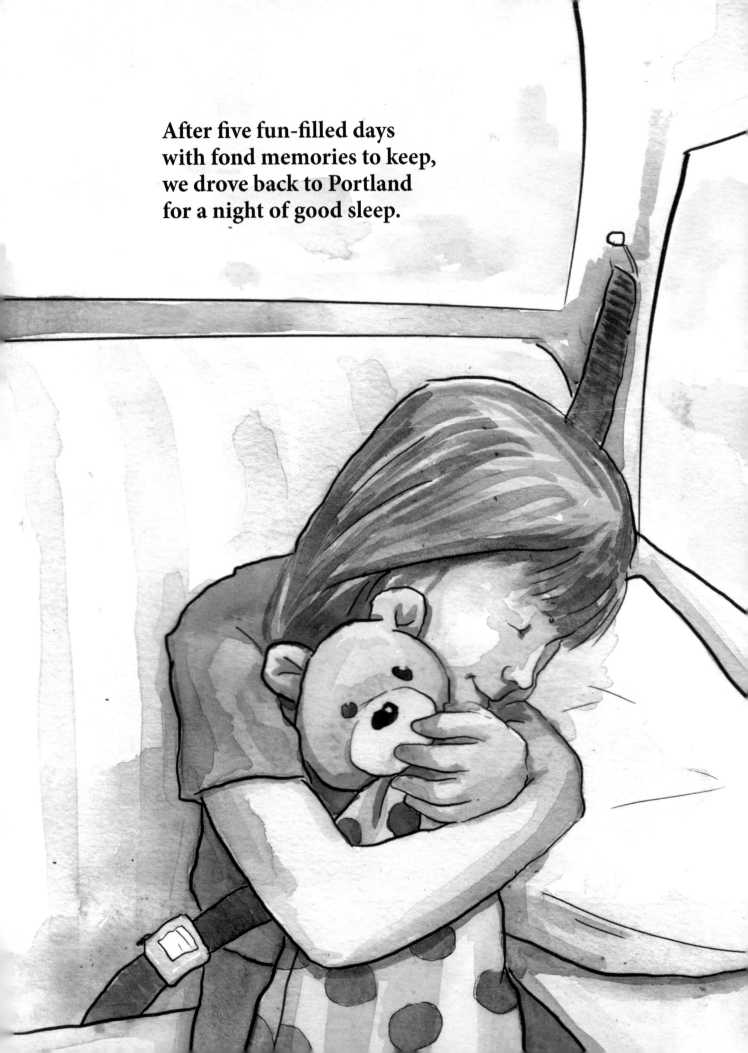

We asked dear sweet Ellie,
"What was your best part?"
"Twirls with Mama and Daddy!"
Such words filled my heart.

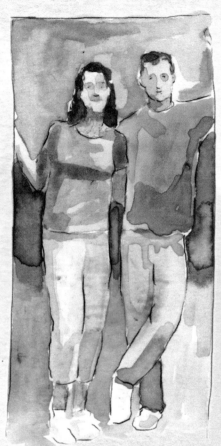

"If I wear my dress, Daddy,
  when the sun lets us see,
  will you dance more with Mama,
  then twirl more with me?"

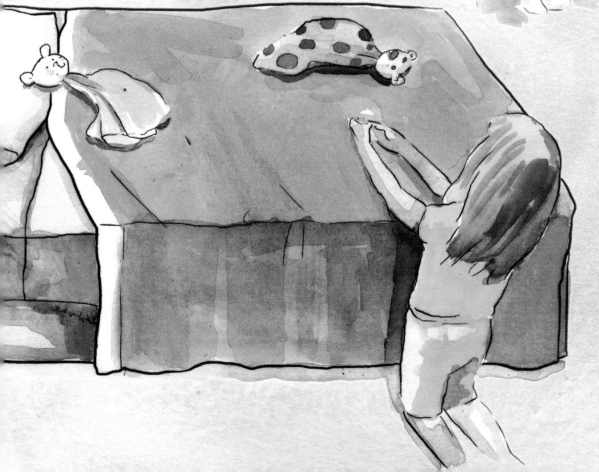

I leaned in much closer and gazed in the face of My Little Love before one last embrace.

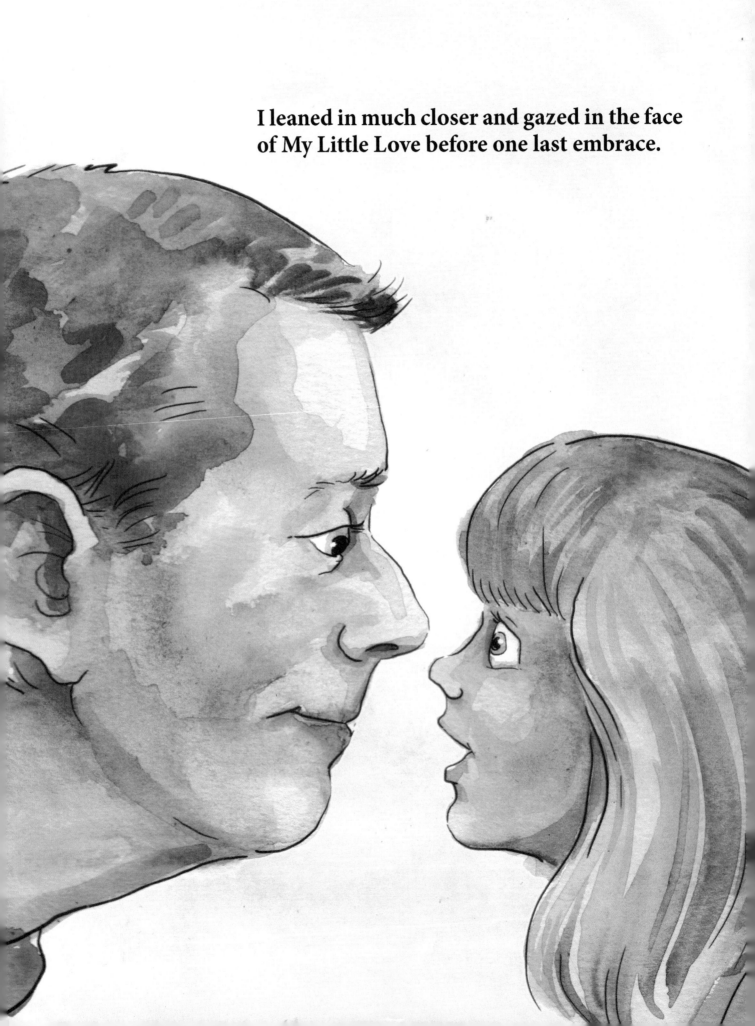

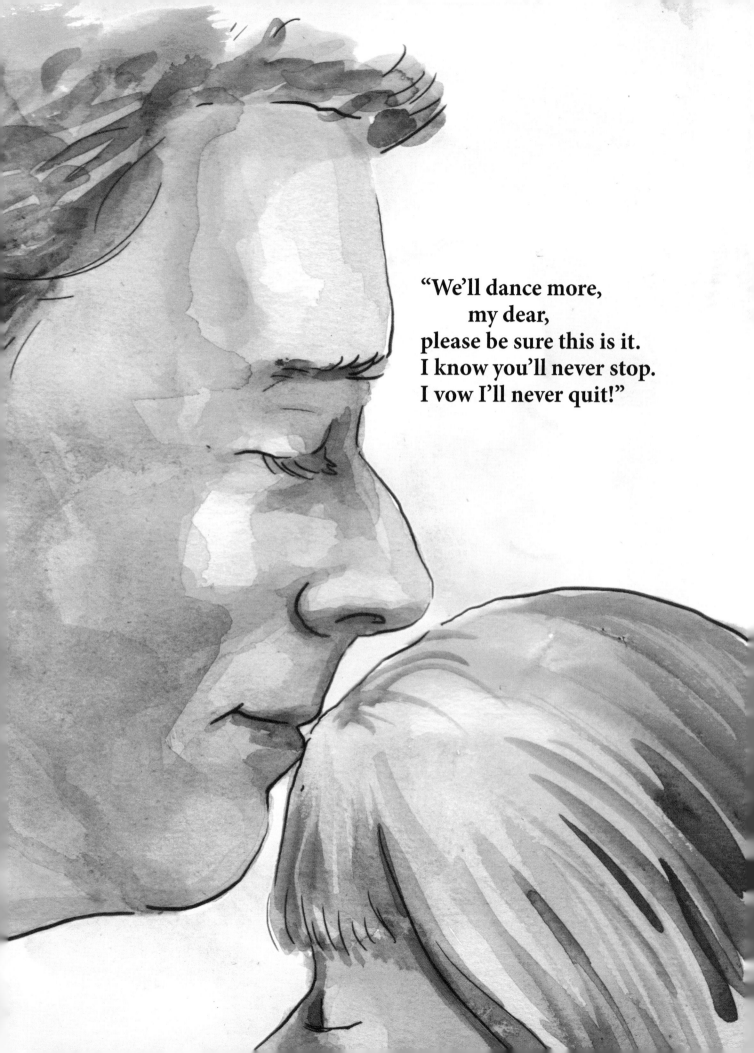

"We'll dance more,
    my dear,
please be sure this is it.
I know you'll never stop.
I vow I'll never quit!"

CPSIA information can be obtained
at www.ICGtesting.com
Printed in the USA
LVIC04n1342230716
497336LV00001B/1